RESTORE AND REJUVENATE

LOOK YOUNGER AND INCREASE YOUR ENERGY WITH RESTORATIVE HEALTH

YOTA PAPAS

ISBN:9781928155263

PUBLISHED BY:
10-10-10 PUBLISHING
MARKHAM, ON
CANADA

Table of Contents

ACKNOWLEDGEMENTS

My deepest thanks to my sisters and family, who supported me through my entire painful emotional breakdown' following my acrimonious divorce and the loss of my children. Thanks, too, to Monica Burton, who helped 'build me back up' when I was at my lowest ebb. My deepest gratitude also goes to Anthony Deavin for 'fixing my back' with a polarity session while I was 'a guinea pig' in a workshop. He gave me back a healthy and flexible back, and helped me avoid an operation. Plus, he has been my lecturer and master, teaching me this wonderful drugless method of healing. Another thank you goes to Brandon Bays for helping me find my way to 'forgiveness through the 'journey' processes and cellular healing.

All these people were Angels in my life. They came along to help me rebuild myself and my life when there seemed to be no hope in sight, as did Andy Harrington (Jet Set Speaker System). Andy has helped me tremendously in gaining my confidence, looking at my life outside the trappings of my 'story' and disconnecting from the pain. He is a true genius in helping you step out of the you that holds you back from progress. Andy, in turn, brought Raymond Aaron into my life and helped 'pen the pain without the animation.'

I would also like to thank Raymond Aaron for giving me the opportunity to spread a little hope to those who wish to get better health and rejuvenate their lives with a drugless method of healing. And, lastly, thanks to my editor, Miriam Cohen, who helped organize my thoughts so clearly.

Thank you to all these people who helped put Humpty together again. Thank you, thank you, thank you all.

FOREWORD

For most people, the daily wear and tear of a busy and often stressful life takes a toll on their health. So do poor eating patterns, processed foods and lack of sleep. It's likely you too often feel drained of energy or out of sorts. Your first inclination may be to grab a caffeine-loaded energy drink or pop a pill, but there are better, drug-free solutions.

One of the most proven of these is Polarity Therapy, which has been helping diagnose and treat fatigue, aches and other ailments since it was founded by chiropractor Dr. Randolph Stone in the early part of the last century. It is an alternative medicine based on principles that have a long history dating back to Hippocrates, the father of modern medicine.

There are many practitioners worldwide, but only a few genuine authorities on the subject. Yota Papas is one of those special experts. She has chosen to share her knowledge and expertise in this easy to understand, incredibly informative new book. Unlike other alternative healers who expect you to work with them on faith alone, Yota explains the scientific principles behind Polar Therapy to help you understand why this therapeutic method works as well as it does.

In the pages that follow, you'll learn about the healing restorative powers of Polarity Therapy and how to start using its practices immediately to help yourself feel better and more grounded. You'll see how Polarity Therapy can improve everything from your balance to your back. Yota Papas will have you feeling healthier and more energetic in no time at all.

Raymond Aaron
#1 NY Times Best Selling Author

INTRODUCTION

"If we could give every individual the right amount of nourishment and exercise, not too little and not too much, we would have found the safest way to health."

- Hippocrates

The human body is a remarkable, fascinating machine. While its functionality is dependent on a multitude of complex internal systems, it can be impressively resilient, enduring and capable of recovering from damage that would cripple other organisms. Properly fueled and maintained, it can continue to work for at least 100 years.

However, like any other complex machine, the human body requires a lot of maintenance in order to run properly. As its guardians, we don't always provide the right type of fuel and often ignore or dismiss the importance of signals from the body (symptoms) telling us to adjust the mix of food, water and oxygen. We also allow too much stress into our lives and don't take the time to gauge the effect of our hurried lifestyles on the physical and psychological health of our bodies.

Over time, our organs and circulatory system suffer. We develop ailments and illnesses that, left untreated, can do real damage long term. In the short term, our bodies stop functioning optimally. We can become sluggish, irregular, lightheaded or exhibit any one of a number of symptoms that make us feel unwell.

It's not surprising, therefore, that the earliest forms of medical science emerged out of a desire to maximize the human body's functional capabilities. One of the earliest and most influential pioneers in this field was the Ancient Greek physician Hippocrates. From his experience and research, Hippocrates developed a broad theory concerning human health that holds true all these centuries later. Specifically, he surmised that our wellness is dependent on the influx and moderation of our energy, or life force.

In the early 20th Century, a chiropractic doctor, Randolph Stone, developed a theory that vindicated and expanded upon Hippocrates' findings. Like Hippocrates, Dr. Stone believed that our physical and emotional wellness is dependent on the influx of energy into our bodies. This belief was largely based on his discovery of the intricate network of electromagnetic fields flowing through our body. From his research, Dr. Stone developed guiding principles for keeping our bodies healthy and functioning properly. His principles for health have been proven time and again since Dr. Stone developed them.

I consider these two men to be the founding fathers of Polarity Therapy, of which I am a strong proponent and practitioner. Having seen and experienced the results of their scientific theories and principles, I became devoted to the field and to sharing their insights with everyone I can. Among the different forms of therapy available, I chose to practice Polarity Therapy in part because it emphasizes the body's natural cycles and healing from within.

Not enough of us take advantage of the body's ability to regulate and heal itself — to rejuvenate, if you will. Our society encourages us to eat the wrong things, take the wrong chemicals, run full speed ahead without taking a breath and, in general, search for the 'magic bullets' that will miraculously cure everything in one dose or less.

You don't have to — and shouldn't — live like that. Thanks to the findings of both Hippocrates and Dr. Stone, the key to living happily and healthily is well within your reach. No longer will you go entire days feeling lethargic and drained without ever knowing why. No longer will you look in the mirror and wonder why that lethargy is reflected on your face and in your eyes. No longer will you spend months experimenting with different diet pills and exotic treatments that are only designed to drain your bank account. It's time for you to take control of your own life, and you can do just that once you recognize that it's all a matter of controlling your energy input and output. Your body is capable of restoring your energy and health with just a little help from you.

Reading this book is a great start. It will explain the scientific tenets upon which Polarity Therapy is based, lay out Dr. Stone's principles in the most simple and clear manner and start you on the way down a healthier and happier path by providing an introduction to breathing and yoga exercises.

And, if you decide to pursue professional help, I hope you will consider Polarity Therapy. It is a gentle approach that marries the best of both Eastern and Western medicine.

Chapter 1
DISCOVERING THE POWER OF
POLARITY THERAPY

"I have stumbled onto a science which blends the old concept of energies in the constitution of man and have linked it with the scientific research of space... as above so below, as within, so without..."

- Dr. Randolph Stone

Polarity Therapy, developed by chiropractor Randolph Stone, DO, DC, ND (among other medical certifications), is based on the understanding that an electromagnetic energy field surrounds the body. That external field is created from within the body, which has an intricate network of electromagnetic fields flowing throughout.

When a body's energy flow is balanced and free of blockages, the body is healthy and functioning at its best. When the body's energy is not flowing optimally, pain and disease result. 'Minor ailments,' like sluggishness or irregularity, are among the symptoms that can alert you to an imbalance.

9

One might say that the Ancient Greek physician Hippocrates is the true founding father of Polarity Theory because of his understanding of the way the body works and the part nutrition plays in getting and staying healthy.Dr. Stone , in turn, developed a discipline of healing based on evaluating and affecting body energy according to movements and magnetic currents.

The Concept of Humors

According to Hippocrates, the human body runs on five substances, called 'humors', each of which represents one of the elements that comprise the universe; a different organ regulates each substance.

Organ	Humor	Element Of the Universe
Liver	Blood	Air
Spleen	Yellow Bile	Fire
Gall Bladder	Black Bile	Earth
Brain & Lungs	Phlegm	Water
Immune System	White Plasma	One's Aura

Hippocrates theorized that every illness or disorder could be explained by a surplus or deficit of one of these substances.

Dr. Stone's Elements

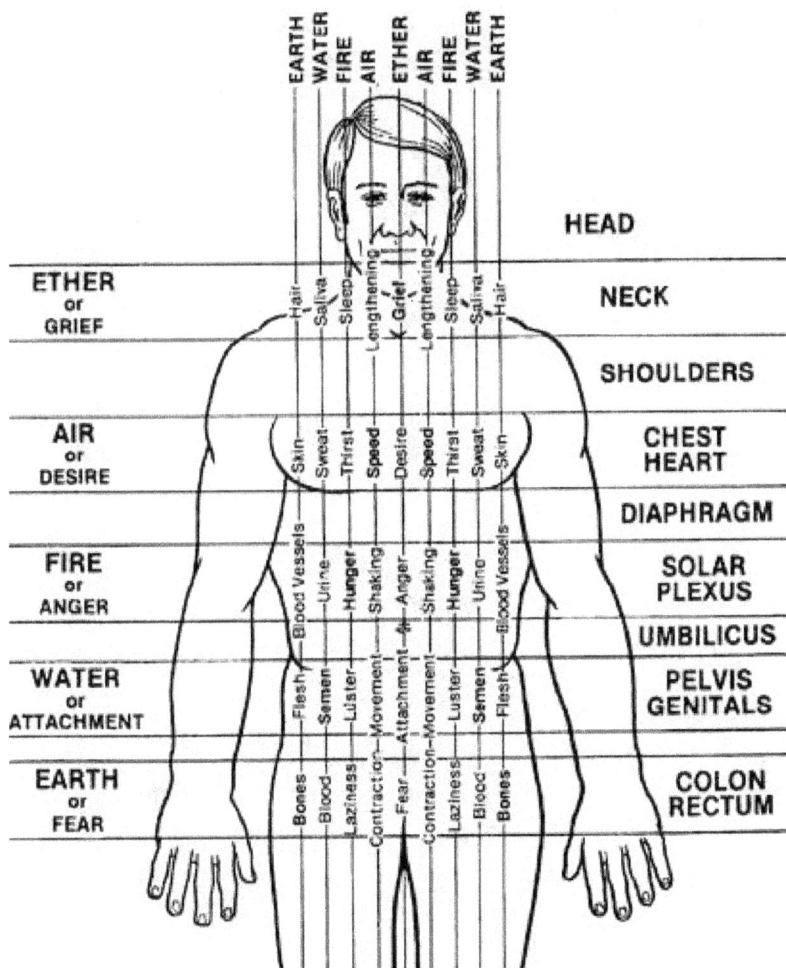

EARTH WATER FIRE AIR ETHER AIR FIRE WATER EARTH

HEAD

ETHER or **GRIEF**

Hair · Saliva · Sleep · Longthening · Grief · Longthening · Sleep · Saliva · Hair

NECK

SHOULDERS

AIR or **DESIRE**

Skin · Sweat · Thirst · Speed · Desire · Speed · Thirst · Sweat · Skin

CHEST HEART

DIAPHRAGM

FIRE or **ANGER**

Blood Vessels · Urine · Hunger · Shaking · Anger · Shaking · Hunger · Urine · Blood Vessels

SOLAR PLEXUS

UMBILICUS

WATER or **ATTACHMENT**

Flesh · Semen · Luster · Movement · Attachment · Movement · Luster · Semen · Flesh

PELVIS GENITALS

EARTH or **FEAR**

Bones · Blood · Laziness · Contraction · Fear · Contraction · Laziness · Blood · Bones

COLON RECTUM

Moderation and Balance

To Hippocrates, good health was all a matter of balance and equilibrium. The concept of opposing forces working together in harmony is a recurring theme in a wide variety of ancient cultures (like the concept of the 'yin' and the 'yang' in Far Eastern philosophy). All over the world, people have viewed the universe as a series of dichotomies and dualities: night and day, dark and light, heat and cold. Hippocrates, however, was one of the first Western thinkers to apply this concept to the field of medicine. To him, the ideas of moderation and balance could easily be implemented to promote healthy living and physical wellness.

Additionally, Hippocrates developed one of the earliest codes of ethics for medical practitioners to follow. He penned the document that we know today as the Hippocratic Oath, which novice physicians are still required to swear upon to this day. Those who take the Oath swear to treat their patients and colleagues as they would their own brothers and sisters, instruct them in the art of healthy living and devote themselves entirely to the protection and maintenance of the well being of others. It was Hippocrates who popularized the notion that, first and foremost, a doctor should do no harm. As you'll see, the same adage applies to each and every one of us.

The Birth of Polarity Therapy

Based on his discovery and mapping of the electromagnetic fields within the body, Dr. Stone developed a method of healing that he called 'Polarity Therapy.' It is based on the idea that positive health is a product of the individual's ability to control and regulate the flow of energy throughout his or her body.

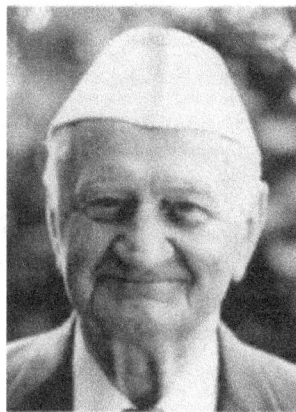

'Polarity Therapy' got its name from the manner in which energy tends to move. The flow of energy is driven by both attractive and repulsive forces, a perpetual system of pushes and pulls. The repulsive forces drive energy out from a central force while the attractive forces draw it back in, maintaining a constant equilibrium.

Again, this can all be traced back to the theories of Hippocrates. The methods employed by Dr. Stone are based on the concept of polarized opposite forces (one attractive, one repulsive). This mirrors Hippocrates' writings concerning the ubiquitous presence of dichotomies and parallel forces in nature. And, again, the Chinese concept of yin and yang represents the same principle.

With respect to breathing, Hippocrates related it to waves lapping in and out of the shore. In turn, Dr. Stone likened breathing to the 'tidal waves' of the sea in terms of their 'timing' and rhythm. As the angry sea is unstable, the calm sea is relaxed and can sometimes be 'still.'

These opposing forces work in harmony, dictating the movement of energy throughout the universe, throughout nature, and throughout our bodies. As a consequence, all of our bodily processes and systems are expressions of that life energy in motion. Good health and the process of healing are effects of the flow of energy maintaining or returning to its natural, default state.

Three Driving Principles

From this theory, Dr. Stone was able to formulate three principles of polarity- based motion, based on three of the four Ancient Greek elements. Each of these principles corresponds to the kinetic properties of its respective element.

According to the Water Principle, energy moves throughout the body via 'long line currents,' which carry energy in and out of the body in the same manner as a body of running water. By contrast, the Fire Principle postulates that energy radiates outward and inward in a spiral-like motion, not unlike the

Three Vibratory Principles in Polarity Therapy

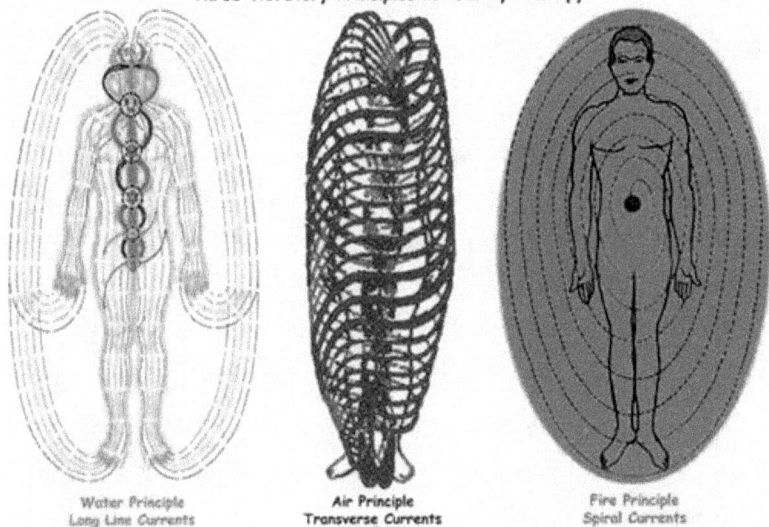

| Water Principle | Air Principle | Fire Principle |
| Long Line Currents | Transverse Currents | Spiral Currents |

manner in which heat radiates outward from a flame. The Air Principle maps out the flow of energy as a series of transverse currents, which swirl in and out of the body at a rapid pace independent of gravity.

While some were initially skeptical of Dr. Stone's theories, he was able to prove that they were, in fact, valid. Early on in his career, he worked extensively with handicapped people, particularly paraplegics and hopeless cases. With his revolutionary therapeutic methods, he was able to lift their spirits, improve their health, and (in rare cases) restore their capacity to walk. The phenomenon of helping the lame walk has been observed and documented for centuries (with the biblical story of the cripple being the most notable example), and Dr. Stone confirmed that this phenomenon is both viable and provable.

How Does Polarity Therapy Work?

A gentle and holistic form of healing, Polarity Therapy puts the principles of Dr. Stone into practice through touch, manipulation, exercise and diet and lifestyle changes. Polarity Therapy is extremely effective in alleviating the ailments that result from an energy imbalance but, unlike traditional medicine, it is useful in both disease prevention and the maintaining of a healthy state.

One of the beautiful things about Polarity Therapy is that a good portion of what it entails is done by you, the patient. Of course, that means you must be willing to make the necessary changes in the way you eat, move and breathe. Of course, once you realize how much better these changes make you feel, you will want to continue with your new and healthier lifestyle.

Chapter 2
TREATING THE COMPLETE NERVOUS SYSTEM

Your entire nervous system plays an integral part in balancing your energy flow. I'm not going to take you through the science in detail at this point. Suffice it to say that each part of the body's nervous system has a role to play. Polarity Therapy focuses on three parts of the nervous system, (The Autonomic, Sympathetic and Parasympathetic Systems), but the other three are complimented by being balanced in a complete session. The Central Nervous System is affected by the Polarity Therapist's work on the Cerebral Spinal Fluid (CSF). Here is a summary that highlights the role each part of your complete nervous system plays in the flow of energy throughout your body:

- The Autonomic Nervous System: Positive Pole
- The Sympathetic Nervous System: Responds to 'fight or flight' situations
- The Parasympathetic Nervous System: Negative Pole
- The Peripheral Nervous System: Controls the fourth and sixth cranial nerves relating to eye movements
- The Central Nervous System: Controlled by the CSF (about which you'll learn more later in this chapter)

- The Enteric Nervous System: Otherwise known as the 'colon,' comes mostly under the Autonomic System

Moderation and the Vagus Nerve

The state of your overall health is, for the most part, dependent on the actions of the vagus nerve. Vital to the process of self-moderation, the nerve is a major conduit of information to and from the brain. Perhaps the longest nerve in the body, it connects the brain with most of your vital organs, allowing the brain to learn about problems in the body and react to correct those problems. In other words, it tells the brain when it needs to moderate the body.

Made up of both motor and sensory fibers, the vagus nerve passes through the neck and thorax to the abdomen, coming into contact with, in part, the voice box, lungs, heart and stomach. It is also called Cranial Nerve X, (it's the 10th Cranial Nerve) or the Wandering Nerve (*vagus* is Latin for 'wandering').

The vagus nerve carries a wide assortment of signals to and from the

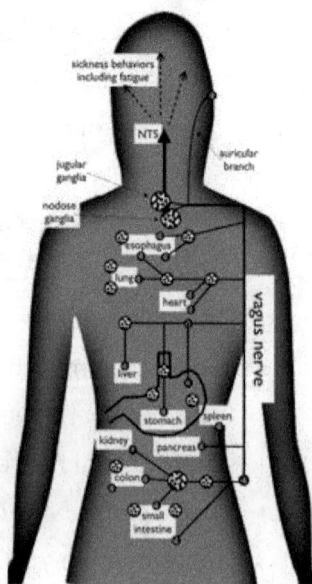

brain. Those signals alert the brain to problems in the various organs of the viscera — that part of the body which is commonly called 'the innards' or the 'guts.' Similar signals traveling along the nerve are responsible for the associated reflex responses in the body.

In simple terms, that means the vagus nerve helps regulate your heartbeat, keeps you breathing, helps your digestive track work properly, contracts stomach and intestinal muscles involved in processing food and transmits chemicals from the brain throughout your body. Part of the information being sent back and forth is about what foods are being digested and what the body is getting out of those foods. The nerve tells the brain when you've eaten too much sugar, protein or fat with the intent of keeping your body moderated.

When something is amiss, it activates the vagus nerve which, in turn, causes the brain to take defensive measures. Those measures are manifested as a number of different psychological and physiological effects. People with overactive vagus nerves frequently suffer from dehydration, irritable bowel syndrome or fainting and dizziness, among other symptoms. These symptoms need to be addressed if you are to regain your healthy state. While treatment may be needed for some of these ailments, others are easily correctable through your own efforts. With that said, doctors have been able to formulate different types of therapy that involve deliberate stimulation of the vagus nerve. Physicians have found that stimulation often serves as an effective treatment for depression due to its tendency to heighten the activity of the nervous system. This form of therapy is also beneficial to patients who have frequent seizures, and some scientists have claimed that it can be used to treat patients with Alzheimer's, frequent migraines and anxiety disorder.

Since the vagus nerve is so powerful and can produce a multitude of effects when activated, it is important to learn to manage it. If you suffer from frequent dizziness, for instance, you may have an overactive vagus nerve, in which case you should consult your physician about the problem as soon as you can. On the other hand, if you frequently feel depressed or lethargic, then your vagus nerve may not be active enough, and you might want to consider vagus stimulation treatment. The important thing is that you know who you are, what your needs are, and how to fulfill them.

It has been noted that some of the greatest 'miracles' have occurred when the vagus nerve is worked on during Polarity treatment. There have been amazing recoveries from brain injuries or trauma, as well as Post Traumatic Stress Disorder (PTSD), because the vagus kicked in and helped activate 'neuroplasticity' (changes in neural pathways and synapses).

The Spine

Your spine is the journal of your whole life. Through Dr. Stone's work and the study ofAsian and other other Oriental methods of healing, as well as his experience as an osteopath and chiropractor, he discovered that manipulating and deeply palpating the spine gives the patient the beneficial effects of working on other channels. In addition, Dr. Stone found that, when working on the front of the body (the 'weaker' part of the anatomy, or the yin), the organs were more likely to 'participate' in the healing process when the equivalent part of the 'tri band' was connected (The body divides parts of the body into sections with equal measures of energy; see illustrations at right and on page 26. On the illustration on page 26, particularly note the white, lighter gray and darker gray sections). For example, if Dr. Stone was working on the 'Fire' element, he would connect to another part of the body with that same element point, and the 'blockage' would clear.

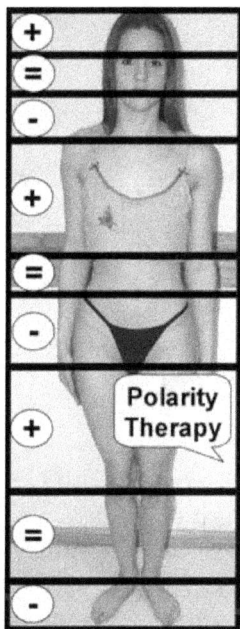

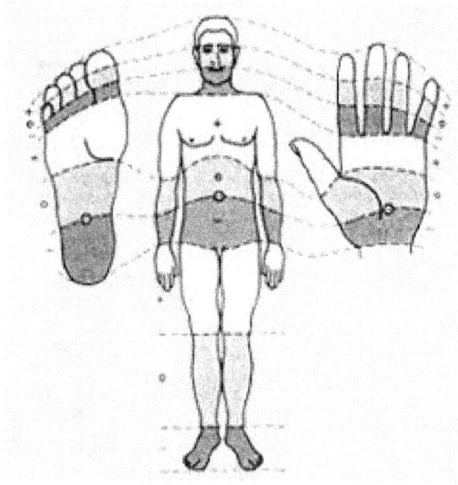

Osteopath John Upledger (the founder of CranioSacral Therapy and author of *CranioSacral Therapy, CranioSacral Therapy II - Beyond The Dura and SomatoEmotional Release and Beyond*) continued Dr. Stone's research in this method of healing. As a paediatrician and osteo surgeon, he found that Cranio Sacral therapy concentrates on the membranes and the CSF surrounding the brain and Spinal cord. As Candace Pert, PhD and author of *Molecules Of Emotion: The Science Behind Mind-Body Medicine* went on to explain, at the most basic level there are two groups of molecules that work together to create emotions: peptides and receptors. She believed that memories are stored in the peptide receptor cells and that emotional release through bodywork is direct evidence of the theory that our cells retain such memories.

Upledger also confirmed that the body stores emotions in the form of 'energy cysts,' which are created when trauma enters the body via a physical or emotional experience. He proved that if the body is placed to mimic' the original position at the time of injury, the body will align the tissues in such a way that it allows the cell memory to escape and dissipate.

CSF

In order to gain control of the electromagnetic fields within your body, you need to understand where they come from, which is the CSF. The bodily fluid enveloping your brain and your spine, CSF is responsible for keeping us alive and healthy in a number of different ways. It acts as a shock absorber, cushioning the brain and the spine from injury. Secondly, it helps circulate nutrients throughout the body while disposing of waste products excreted from the body. Many diseases of the nervous system can and have been diagnosed after examining the condition of the CSF, making it a reliable indicator of your body's overall health.

Chapter 4
INVOKING THE PRINCIPLES OF
POLARITY THERAPY

Now that you know the principles of Polarity Therapy, you can begin to understand how it works on a philosophical and ideological level. Doing so will help you put its teachings and practices to use to improve your health and, subsequently, your quality of life and longevity.

In order to do that, we need to revisit the teachings of Hippocrates. Hippocrates was, first and foremost, a contributor to the Greek field of medical science. However, he also played a major role in the development of Greek thought. And Greek thought is very powerful indeed.

Do No Harm

As I mentioned earlier in this book, the first principle of Hippocrates' teachings is, above all else, to *do no harm*. This is such a powerful principle that it has lasted through the centuries as evidenced by the fact that new doctors still have to take an oath to promise that they will only act in a way that is optimal to the health of their patients. However, the *do no harm* principle does not only apply to doctors and physicians; it applies to *you*.

While the doctor's job is to help you and offer you advice, doctors cannot take care of patients who are unwilling to take care of themselves. And, sometimes, taking care of yourself involves seriously considering the pros and cons of a doctor's advice and learning about other treatment modalities, like Polarity Therapy. This is not to say that what we now call 'traditional' or Western medicine is to be avoided. Rather, that it is but one of several possible treatment modes which can be used jointly for the most positive outcomes in terms of your own health.

First and foremost, you can follow the principle of doing no harm to yourself by making wise, considered lifestyle choices. You don't need to go to the extreme — that is, turn your life and your eating habits upside down — in order to be healthier. In many ways, this is about having common sense.

Plus, making wise choices for yourself will allow you to extend your healing prowess to others, healing them by education or by deed. By helping yourself, you will enable yourself to help others, and to help others help themselves. Each of us can make an enormous difference in terms of how we and the ones we care about feel on a daily basis.

Know Your Limits

Proper nutrition and hydration are essential for healing and optimal health. In fact, the adage "you are what you eat" is actually a sound piece of advice. Dr. Stone recommended a vegetarian diet of organic fresh fruits and vegetables (in season being the best option), and encouraged people to eat few or no processed foods. As is now commonly recommended by nutritionists worldwide, Dr. Stone emphasized eating whole grains instead of flour, staying away from food cooked in oil and limiting alcohol, coffee, soda and sugar consumption. In this way, he was at the forefront of recommending low glycemic index foods. Likewise, he was among the first — if not *the* first — to recognize that there are good fats and carbohydrates as well as bad ones.

(Alfalfa sprouts, fenugreek, mung beans and lentils are also healthy food choices because they are low in sugars, high in fiber vitamins and minerals; they are generally full of goodness.)

As you may have noticed, the theories of both Hippocrates and Dr. Stone are largely based around the concept of moderation. The influx of humors into your body should never be greater or less than the excretion of said humors. In a modern scientific context, this means monitoring the vitamins, minerals, fats, sugars and carbohydrates you take in every day. The levels of each substance in your body should always be kept at a medium level: not too low, not too high. This is a much safer and sound way of approaching food than those fad diets that encourage you to eat only protein (more about that later in the next paragraph) or one particular food, like grapefruit.

Also note that this applies to *all* substances, including the ones that we normally view in a negative light. Take fat, for instance. Most of us are concerned with limiting or even eliminating our fat intake, but fat actually plays a vital role in the way our bodies function. Fat is the body's portable grocery, providing us with an easily accessible source of energy. It also serves to protect us from injury by cushioning our bones. Obviously, it can be harmful if we take in too much of it, but it would be just as unwise to avoid it at all costs.

By the same token, substances that we typically see as beneficial can be harmful if our intake of them is too great. Protein is a perfect example. In acceptable doses, it can provide you with the energy you need and help your muscles recover from damage. But, increasing your protein intake without increasing the number of calories you ingest accordingly (i.e., from non-protein foods) may put your bodily systems under excessive stress. It can also lead to the buildup of toxic ketones (molecules generated during the metabolism of fat), which, in turn, can cause dizziness, dehydration and other health problems.

Obviously, our bodies need protein, but it is important to make sure that you're not taking in any less or any more than you need.

Again, the key is moderation and the finer essences are the energy principles in food. That is the foundation of our health which, in return, gives us the energy we need.

Stay Hydrated

Proper hydration is necessary in order to keep just about every part of the body functioning properly. Water holds the cells of the body together and is crucial to energy production at the cellular level. Hydrolysis (the splitting of the water molecule into hydrogen and oxygen) releases water and generates energy that helps produce adenosine triphosphate (ATP) — a major source of energy stored in the body. Additionally, the brain is mostly comprised of water (85% fully hydrated), and the energy for many of its parts comes from water.

Neurotransmission (the transmission of a signal along a nerve) is also heavily dependent upon water intake and, in fact, chronic nerve pain is often the result of chronic dehydration. It is just as often easily addressed by significantly increasing the amount of water you consume on a regular basis. Furthermore, dehydration of the lungs is a causative factor in respiratory diseases and produces stress in the body. It also changes the balance of amino acids and, as a result, can contribute to DNA errors during cell division. That can lead to cell mutation and major diseases like cancer.

Hydration is also critical for regulating your metabolism. Dehydration of the cells causes or contributes to all the metabolic problems in the body. In particular, it has a dramatic effect on the metabolism of sugar, detoxification of the body and the immune system. Dehydration can also affect your emotions, and keeping the body effectively hydrated eliminates the production of and removes free radicals faster than any other therapy, thus making it unnecessary to take antioxidant supplements. Proper hydration can even have a profoundly beneficial effect on the look of your skin, effectively taking years off your appearance.

Although there has been a lot written about the importance of staying hydrated, most people still live under the misunderstanding that any liquid they drink will suffice. Not drinking enough pure fluids, specifically water without additives like coffee and cola, can result in cellular dehydration. Soda, tea, coffee and even some herbal teas contain caffeine or other substances that function like caffeine; that's a problem because caffeine is a dehydrating agent. So is alcohol. They both increase kidney function and, when not balanced by a sufficient amount of 'straight' water, can actually cause damage to the tissues and cells in your body.

Use Natural Remedies

Every year, food and drug industries make millions of dollars from naïve consumers who are looking for quick, easy ways to resolve their health problems. Do *not* become one of these people. It can be quite tempting to try the 'magic bullet,' but it is important to remember that the manufacturers and marketers of these products don't have your best interests at heart. The companies who make these artificial slimming agents and so-called 'miracle drugs' are only concerned with squeezing as much money out of you as they can.

In reality, these drugs only serve to upset the long-term balance of your humors (Hippocrates) or elements (Dr. Stone), not to mention how they can contaminate your CSF or overtax your heart, while providing little more than short-term relief, if that. If you truly want to balance your humors, do it naturally instead of trying to take shortcuts (see Chapter 4).

Exercise

Movement and associated nerve messages optimize brain function. Polarity yoga exercises are designed to affect our energy and physiologic functioning in a positive manner. They energize you and make you feel more relaxed and grounded at the same time. (See Chapter 6 for specific exercises.)

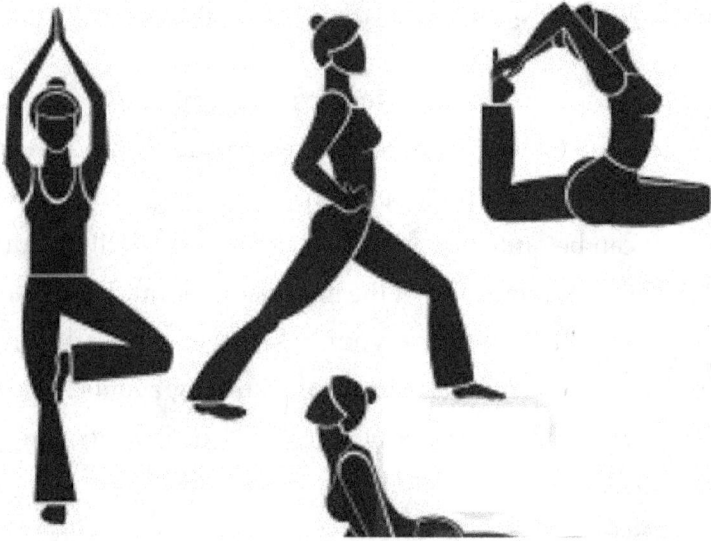

Manipulation

In addition to stretching and moving, physically pressing on specific body points is an integral part of Polarity Therapy. It is highly effective at releasing stuck patterns that block the energy flow from moving harmoniously (and thus causing pain and discomfort). Sometimes, simply placing hands on the body is sufficient to allow the energy to do its work and help the connective tissue release the discomfort causing the pain/problem/emotion. Of course, it takes a trained Polarity Therapist to diagnose where the problems are and to deliver the appropriate touching treatment. There are three different 'pressure touches' a practitioner uses, and those pressure touches are applied according to the treatment.

Chapter 5
PUTTING STONE'S PRINCIPLES TO WORK

As a sort of corollary to the 'do no harm' principle, Dr. Stone postulated "when a doctor cannot do good, he must be kept from doing harm." By this, he meant that if a doctor is not confident that he is capable of prescribing a treatment that will help his patient, he should abstain from prescribing any treatment at all. After all, if the doctor cannot be sure whether his treatment will improve the patient's health, then logically, he cannot be sure whether his treatment will worsen his patient's health. (Of course, not all doctors practice this principle of Dr. Stone's and, to be fair, the area can be a very gray one as new treatments are discovered, especially for grave medical disorders like cancer.)

Like the original 'do no harm' principle, this one is just as relevant to you as it is to licensed doctors. As I've said before, all too often people are quick to jump on a revolutionary miracle drug or a new fad diet before they have a clear understanding of what the effects of those things will be. Every day, we see advertisements for new diet pills and receive spam emails from people who claimed to have, "dropped two dress sizes in three weeks just by following one simple rule! Click the link below to find out more!"

For the most part, the credibility of these claims is dubious, and you shouldn't rely on them being true. Always, *always, always* do your research before adopting any significant change in diet or lifestyle. Nowhere is this truer than when it comes to these 'hype' drugs. Make sure you know *exactly* how the new treatment is supposed to work, and whether it can adequately fulfill your needs. For instance, if a drug is only designed to lower cholesterol levels, then it would not be of any use to you unless you have unusually high cholesterol. And, don't take thyroid medicine just to lose weight. Remember, if it sounds too good to be true, it probably is.

In most cases, it's preferable to avoid those kinds of commercial treatments altogether. 'Trendy' drugs and diets are often backed by giant corporations, and corporations generally aren't concerned with whether or not your long-term health actually improves. On top of that, most of the treatments they 'prescribe' involve the ingestion of artificial, man-made drugs and stimulants. At this point, it should come to no surprise that, according to Dr. Stone, the best remedies are taken directly from the natural world. As he put it, "natural forces within us are the true healers of disease."

Breathing

"Practicing regular, mindful breathing can be calming and energizing and can even help with stress-related health problems ranging from panic attacks to digestive disorders."

— Andrew Weil, M.D.

The system that is most directly responsible for energy input and output is, of course, the respiratory system. Regardless of the type of therapy you are employing, learning how to breathe properly — fully filling and emptying your lungs — is one of the most important lessons to be learned.

The power and influence of your breathing is enormous. Breathing in is, after all, the first action we take upon being born, and breathing out is the last action we take before we die. Because we perform it instinctually, most people never consciously think about the action of breathing, let alone monitor or regulate their breathing patterns.

The way you breathe has an undeniable effect on your physiology, your mood and your stress level. When you don't breathe to the fullest, your lungs don't take in enough oxygen, which means that you have less than optimal oxygen levels in your bloodstream. That can have both immediate and long-term effects on your heart. Additionally, insufficient oxygen in the bloodstream keeps the other organs in your body from functioning properly. Many of the ailments people suffer from can be cured or mitigated simply by learning to breathe fully and in rhythm. Controlling your own breathing can help calm you down when overly anxious or excited, help alleviate some dizziness or lightheadedness and elevate you out of minor depression. It also helps circulatory problems.

Therefore, in order to maximize your body's health, you must learn to control your breathing instead of letting your breathing control you. One way to promote healthy breathing is to partake in a series of breathing exercises daily. Here are the three I recommend for beginners. Note how important it is in these exercises to empty your lungs completely. (For many people with respiratory problems, not letting all the air in their lungs out is the biggest problem they have — and it is so easily correctable through exercises like these.)

Breathing Exercises

4-7-8 Breath

The '4-7-8 Breath,' practiced and taught by Dr. Andrew Weil, is proven to be an effective way to promote good breathing habits. It helps you control the pace of both your inhale and exhale, and tends to have a soothing effect on the brain. The exercise is easy to learn, requires no equipment of any sort and can be done anywhere. While it also can be done in any position, those who are just beginning to learn the exercise should perform it with their back straight.

1. Place the tip of your tongue just behind your upper front teeth, and keep it there.
2. Exhale through your mouth. You should be making a 'whoosh' sound.
3. Close your mouth and count to four while you slowly inhale the breath back through your nose.
4. Hold that breath for seven counts, and release it for eight counts.

Keep in mind that you need to keep your tongue behind your front teeth at all times during this exercise.

Belly Breath

This breath, adapted from yoga, is designed to cleanse the lungs, increase your energy level and relieve stress.

1. Lie down on the floor, flat on your back. If you want, you can place cushions under your neck and legs to reduce the strain on those areas.
2. Place both of your hands on your tummy, just below

your ribs. Your middle fingers should be just barely touching each other.

3. Take a deep breath in and slowly let it out.

If you are doing this exercise correctly, your belly should expand and push your fingers apart while you breathe in. This is an indication that you are breathing from your diaphragm, resulting in a truly deep breath. Get into the habit of breathing from your diaphragm instead of your chest, as doing so increases your lungs' maximum capacity.

Alternate Nostril Breathing

Also known as 'Nadi Shodhana,' this breathing technique is often used by yoga practitioners as a way of uniting the left and right sides of the brain, thereby achieving mental as well as physical balance.

1. Cover up your right nostril and inhale deeply through your left.
2. As soon as you've taken in as much air as you can, cover up the left nostril and let the air out through the right.
3. Repeat this pattern between five and ten times for each nostril, or until you feel the air freely flowing as your breath travels throughout your body with no obstructions.

You Feel As You Eat

The generation of electromagnetic energy *outside* your body is a result of the circulation of energy *inside* your body (which can be attributed to the CSF). Thus, keeping your energy levels high is a matter of keeping your CSF clean and healthy.

How, you may ask, does one do that? Well, it's all a matter of what you take in. In large part, this is probably not new information to you. Many healers, homeopaths, dieticians and other leaders in the field of nutrition have been getting the word out that healthy is as healthy eats. In some ways, all are advocating a way of taking in nutrition that represents a return to a healthier past — before processed and 'chemicalized' food became the norm.

This is especially true when it comes to Polarity Therapy and energy healing. According to Dr. Stone, your diet plays an instrumental role in the management of your body's vital energy. As such, he also gave extensive dieting advice to his patients. This is another aspect of medicine that he (and many others in other fields of healing) borrowed from Hippocrates, who instructed his patients to, "Let food be thy medicine and medicine be thy food."

Dr. Stone's recommendations on nutrition can be condensed into two habits that have been scientifically proven to be crucial for overall health:

- **Eat a good deal of fresh fruit and vegetables** (ideally five servings a day). Make sure that they're organically farmed and grown, so you can avoid infecting your CSF with artificial preservatives, pesticides and growth hormones.
- **In general, stay away from processed or pre-cooked meals.** In today's society, it can be difficult to stay away from processed foods entirely, but do the best you can to avoid them. Canned, microwaveable and frozen dinners, while convenient, do not do your body any favors. Neither do white bread and flour-laden products.

In fact, Stone theorized that a great number of illnesses and diseases could be traced back to the consumption of these meals. "There are over fifteen hundred diseases," he said, "and only the transgression of nature is the cause of most of them. Therefore, by removing the cause, a multitude of symptoms will disappear." You may be amazed by the number of physical issues you can eliminate just by changing your diet.

The Polarity Diet

People often worry that eating healthy can be boring. Not so. There are a wide variety of foods to choose from:

Beans:	Burdock	Turnip and greens
Sprouted Only	Cabbage, all	Watercress
Aduki	Carrot	Zucchini
Mung	Cauliflower	**Fruits:**
Nuts and Seeds:	Celery	Apple
Sprouted Only	Chives	Apricot
Alfalfa	Collards	Blackberry
Almonds	Cucumber	Cantaloupe
Fenugreek	Eggplant	Cherry
Radish	Endive	Fig
Red Clover	Escarole	Grape
Sunflower	Fennel	Grapefruit
Grains:	Green Beans	Huckleberry
Sprouted Only	Kale	Kumquat
Amaranth	Kelp	Lemon
Buckwheat	Kohlrabi	Lime
Millet	Leeks	Mango
Quinoa	Lettuce	Nectarine
Oil:	Mustard greens	Orange
Flax Oil	Okra	Papaya
Olive Oil	Onion	Pear
Young Greens:	Parsley	Peach
Buckwheat	Peas, fresh	Pineapple
Barley	Peppers	Pomegranate
Sunflower	Rutabaga	Raspberry
Wheat	Spinach	Strawberry
Vegetables:	Summer squash	Tangerine
Beets and Greens	Swiss chard	Watermelon
Broccoli	Tomato	

Source: *Esoteric Anatomy*, Bruce Burger, Richard Gordon and Mathaji Vanamali, Sep 11, 1998

It should be noted, however, that no two bodies respond the same way to certain foodstuffs. Food that may have no noticeable effect on one person may cause another person to feel nauseous and lethargic. Therefore, Dr. Stone advised you *not* to change your diet if the food you take in is not causing any noticeable health problems. (This is a very realistic and practical approach that most of us in today's world can appreciate.)

However, if you notice yourself suffering from frequent aches, pains, drowsiness, or a general deficiency of energy, then your diet is more than likely the root of it. This could mean that your best option is adding more whole grains to your diet, cutting out carbs, or trying a combination of herbal supplements — in other words, whatever you believe will promote your body's healing. In sum, the best way to keep your CSF flowing is to cut out artificial, processed food, soda, sugary rich foods that are bad for you, over-the-counter drugs and recreational drugs as they only work to impede the flow of energy throughout your body. Restrict yourself to natural cures and remedies and freshly juiced vegetables and fruit. When you can afford it, buy organic food from your local health food store and, just to be on the safe side, check the label on each product to make sure that it's free of glutens and artificial preservatives and your vegetables / fruits free of heavy pesticides.

If you do eat meat, fish or poultry make sure you know about how that animal was raised, especially what foods it was given. Look for animals who have been given organic feed because it must be free of animal by-products, antibiotics, hormones or genetically altered grains.

Although Western medicine has its uses and provides some relief from symptoms when and where necessary, it is much more logical to prevent any disease with nutrition and 'mindful' living by educating ourselves in the basics of hygiene and health.

Natural Cures and Remedies

Eliminating toxins from your body on a regular basis is critical to maintaining your health and wellbeing. Body cleansing, also known as detoxing, usually involves at least a few days of a liquid or all vegetable diet. It is highly effective and safe to do on a regular basis. A similar process, called a Liver Flush, helps keep the liver and gallbladder 'squeaky clean.' A combination of juices, Epsom salts (magnesium sulphate), oils, selected herbs and enzymes, the Liver Flush is usually done for two to three days at a time. Practitioners often suggest it be done twice a year. Your skin also plays a huge part in the detoxification process. Soaps, antiperspirants, synthetic fibers and skin creams can leave behind toxins that get under your skin and cause a variety of conditions. Those same toxins also have a detrimental effect on the fluid that flows through your lymphatic system.

Dry skin brushing is an excellent technique for removing these toxins. All you need is a soft bristled brush with a long handle. In addition to removing dead skin and unblocking your pores, skin brushing helps 'drain' and cleanses the lymphatic system, energizes your body and increases circulation. Plus, removing toxins this way actually reduces the amount of toxins that your liver, lungs and kidneys must handle.

Herbs

Naturally grown herbs, in their original, unadulterated form, can be used to treat almost any ailment. Here are a few that you may want to add to your garden in the near future:

Ginkgo

Ginkgo is a non-flowering plant that was originally cultivated in China thousands of years ago. After it was discovered by European botanists, it quickly attained worldwide popularity due to its resilience and medicinal qualities.

The health benefits of ginkgo are well documented. As proven by several scientific studies, ginkgo can dramatically improve one's memory, concentration and problem solving abilities. Its cognitive benefits have also allowed doctors to use it to treat dementia and Alzheimer's patients. The other documented medical uses of ginkgo include the improvement of blood flow and treatment of respiratory disorders such as asthma.

However, ginkgo should only be consumed in moderation. It can be toxic if consumed in large quantities since its seeds carry a potentially deadly neurotoxin (appropriately called *ginkgotoxin*). Ginkgotoxin has the potential to cause seizures, convulsions, unconsciousness, and, in rare cases, death.

Ginseng

Ginseng is a plant found in North America and East Asia. The dried root of ginseng is available at most health food stores. For centuries, it has been used to fulfill a variety of different medical purposes as it can function as a stimulant, aphrodisiac, brain booster and a treatment for erectile dysfunction. It can also lower one's blood sugar levels, which makes it particularly useful to those with type I or type II diabetes. Due to its versatility, it is frequently used in commercial energy drinks and sports beverages.

Like ginkgo, ginseng should be consumed responsibly. The overuse of ginseng can result in nervousness, insomnia, nausea or dizziness. It also makes the heart beat faster. For these reasons, it would be wise to consult your physician before deciding if ginseng is right for you. When you do, remember to mention if you are already taking other herbs or natural remedies that act as a stimulant.

Echinacea

Echinacea is a flowering plant native to North America. Since its discovery, the plant has been cultivated primarily for its beneficial effects on the immune system. By increasing your immune response, echinacea helps to fight off illnesses like the common cold and ward off infections. It also relieves pain and, in some cases, can also be used as a laxative, helping expel toxins from the body.

Fortunately, there are no significant risks associated with the consumption of echinacea. While there have been some cases of people experiencing nausea and stomach pain after ingesting the plant, these side effects are rare and easily reversible.

Guarana

Guarana is a climbing plant commonly found in South America, particularly in the Amazon Basin. It is named after the Guaraní tribe, which cultivated the crop for centuries before introducing it to European colonists. Due to its high concentration of caffeine, it is popularly used as a stimulant to improve attention and alertness. Guarana has also been shown to improve memory.

As far as we know, there are no risks or adverse side effects associated with guarana. However, it has been observed to induce weight loss by acting as an appetite suppressant, so it should be taken with caution (especially if you are considerably underweight). Additionally, people with heart conditions should be careful not to ingest too much caffeine.

Oregano

Oregano is a respected 'functional food' because of its nutritional, antioxidant and disease-preventing properties. The herb, whose name means 'delight of the mountains' in Greek, is native to the Mediterranean region. It is an excellent source of minerals like potassium, calcium, manganese, iron, and magnesium. Potassium is an important component of cell and body fluids that helps control heart rate and blood pressure caused by high sodium. Manganese and copper are used by the body as co-factors for the antioxidant enzyme superoxide dismutase. Iron helps prevent anemia. Magnesium and calcium are important minerals for bone metabolism.

Rhodiola

This incredible herb is reported to have amazing properties for the treatment of cancer, depression, diabetes, hearing loss and immune disorders. (A range of antioxidant compounds has been identified in Rhodiola rosea and related species; significant free-radical scavenging activity has been demonstrated for alcohol and water extracts of rhodiola.)

Cancer: Rhodiola has been shown to increase anti-tumour activity by increasing the body's resistance to toxins. Russian researchers have reported that the oral administration of rhodiola inhibited tumour growths in rats by 39% and decreased metastasis by 50%. It improved urinary tissue and immunity in patients with bladder cancer. In other experiments with various types of cancer, including adenocarcinomas, the use of extracts of rhodiola rosea resulted in significant increased survival rate. Rhodiola rosea might be useful in conjunction with some pharmaceutical anti-tumour agents.

Immune System Ailments: Rhodiola both stimulates and protects the immune system by reinstating homeostasis (metabolic balance) in the body. It also increases the natural killer cells (NK) in the stomach and spleen. This action may be due to its ability to normalise hormones by modulating the release of glucocorticoid into the body.

Depression: In animal studies, extracts of rhodiola seem to enhance the transport of serotonin precursors, tryptophan, and 5-hydroxytryptophan into the brain. Serotonin is a widely studied brain neurotransmitter chemical that is involved in many functions, including smooth muscle contraction, temperature regulation, appetite, pain perception, behaviour, blood pressure and respiration.

When balanced, serotonin imparts a sense of contentment and mental ease. On the other hand, too little or too much serotonin has been linked to various abnormal mental states such as clinical depression. Thus, rhodiola has been used by Russian scientists alone or in combination with antidepressants to boost one's mental state; this is a boon in countries and seasons where one is deprived of adequate sun over prolonged periods. This leads to a condition known as Seasonal Affective Disorder (SAD), common to Northern European countries.

Other Benefits: Rhodiola has many other benefits including its ability to improve hearing, regulate blood sugar levels for diabetics and protect the liver from environmental toxins. It has also been shown to activate the lipolytic processes (fat breakdown) and mobilise lipids from adipose tissue to the natural fat burning system of your body for weight reduction. Rhodiola can also enhance thyroid function (without causing hyperthyroidism) and thymus gland function. Plus, it can protect or delay involution that occurs with aging. It can also improve your adrenal gland reserves without causing hypertrophy. Throughout the years, it has shown to improve erectile dysfunction and/or premature ejaculation in men and normalises their prostatic fluid.

Rosemary

Like rhodiola, rosemary is known as a preventive and treatment for a number of significant health issues.

Cancer Prevention: Rosemary contains carnosol, which has been found in studies to be a potent anti-cancer compound. Researchers have had promising results against breast cancer, prostate cancer, colon cancer, leukemia and skin cancer. In one study, researchers gave powdered rosemary to rats for two weeks and found that it reduced the binding of the carcinogen given to the rats by 76%. It also significantly inhibited the formation of breast tumours.

Memory: Rosemary has long been believed to have memory-enhancing properties. In 1529, a herbal book recommended taking rosemary for "weakness of the brain." Today, research has found that rosemary contains a carnosic acid, which has neuroprotective properties that researchers believe may protect against Alzheimer's disease, as well as the normal memory loss that happens with aging.

Remarkably, even the smell of rosemary has been found to improve memory. Test subjects in cubicles were given essential oil of rosemary to smell, and they had better quality of memory and better overall memory than the control group (though their speed of memory was slower compared to the control group).

Migraines: Rosemary has been a popular natural migraine remedy for centuries. To use the herb for this purpose, boil some rosemary in a large pot of water and pour it into a bowl. Place a towel over your head and lean over the pot to inhale the steam for about ten minutes. Because smelling rosemary has been found to improve memory and mood, this method may also help with memory function and put you in a better state of mind.

Bay Leaf

A powerful diabetes treatment, bay leaf is known for its speed of relief. A study conducted by Abdulrahim Aljamal, PhD at the Department of Medical Technology at Zarqa Private University in Jordan, showed that all patients who consumed bay leaves experienced significant reductions in plasma glucose levels in less than one month's time. Further, a dose of one to three grams of ground bay leaf given daily to subjects with type II diabetes created important reductions in blood glucose, cholesterol and triglyceride levels.

Sage

Sage herb parts, whether fresh or dried, are rich sources of minerals like potassium, zinc, calcium, iron, manganese, copper, and magnesium. As mentioned earlier, potassium is an important component of cell and body fluids, which helps control heart rate and blood pressure. Manganese is used by the body as a co-factor for the antioxidant enzyme superoxide dismutase. In terms of the herb's medical properties, the essential oil obtained from sage has been found to have acetylcholinesterase (AChE) enzyme inhibition activities, resulting in increased AChE levels in the brain. AChE improves concentration and may play a role in the treatment methods for memory loss associated with diseases like Alzheimer's.

Thyme

Thyme is packed with minerals and vitamins that are essential for optimum health. Its leaves are one of the richest sources of potassium, iron, calcium, manganese, magnesium, and selenium. Potassium is an important component of cell and body fluids that helps controlling heart rate and blood pressure. Manganese is used by the body as a co-factor for the antioxidant enzyme superoxide dismutase. Iron is required for red blood cell formation.

The herb is also a rich source of many important vitamins such as B-complex vitamins, beta carotene, vitamin A, vitamin K, vitamin E, vitamin C and folic acid.

Using Herbs Safely

Just like any other form of medicine —natural or otherwise — you need to understand what the herbs you take are meant to do, whether they are appropriate for you and how they might interact with other medications and herbs you are already using. Follow these guidelines before taking any herb:

- Research its effects and determine whether it can fulfill what you need at this very moment. If you cannot be sure if its effects are beneficial, you should not be taking it at all. Remember: if you cannot do good, prevent yourself from doing harm.
- Check to see if there are any adverse side effects.
- Consult your physician beforehand to make sure that the herb is compatible with your physiology. In other words, make sure that you don't have any allergies to the herb in question and that your body won't have any other adverse reaction to it. And, again , make sure that your physician knows about all the medications and herbs you are already taking. It's all a matter of being aware of what you're giving your body at any given time.

- Grow your own herbs if you possibly can but, if you cannot, make sure to buy them from reputable health shops and supermarkets to make sure they have all the properties they claim to have.

Chapter 6
YOGA, MEDITATION AND RELAXATION

This chapter will help you develop your ability to relax. In regards to your health, this is one of the most valuable skills to have. As mentioned before, it is important to keep all of your bodily functions running at a moderate level. This includes your levels of stress and anxiety. People who have trouble managing their tension and adrenaline levels tend to suffer from a variety of different health problems, including high blood pressure, weakened immune systems and sleep deprivation.

Thankfully, moderating your stress levels is simply a matter of exacting control over your body, and there are several techniques that will help you do that. One of those techniques is the Ancient Hindu art of yoga.

Polarity Yoga

One of the oldest holistic healing systems in the world, yoga is a remarkable help in allowing the body to heal itself. It creates an inner sense of peace and stretches and moves the body while maximizing the intake and release of oxygen during breathing.

Colloquially, the word 'yoga' often refers to a series physical exercises designed to improve one's balance and flexibility. In reality, however, the art of yoga encompasses far more than just holding poses for a set amount of time. Yoga is a way of life, a spiritual philosophy designed to guide us toward a higher plane of existence. It was first developed in ancient India as a way of maintaining physical and mental peace.

Like Hippocrates, the originators of yoga valued the idea of maintaining equilibrium. The primary goal of the yoga practitioner (or 'yogi') is to attain evenness of mind, body and spirit while moving towards a state of peaceful, untainted bliss. The idea of achieving physiological and spiritual balance is a key part of the philosophy of yoga.

It should be noted that there *is* a major physical aspect of yoga, and the exercises are a good way to begin the path towards spiritual enlightenment as well as the manifesting of physical health.

Exercises

Self-help is an important concept in Polarity Therapy, and exercise is one crucial way to take charge of your health physically, mentally and emotionally. Polarity Therapy exercises facilitate the movement of energy in both in and between the body and the mind. The goals are improved posture, a relaxed mind and an integrated understanding of the mind-body connection.

Here are some simple exercises to get you started. The movements involved may remind you of traditional Hatha Yoga but are easier to do!

The Tree Pose

The tree pose involves balancing yourself on just one leg. It's not as difficult as it sounds!

1. First, shift your weight onto your left foot.
2. Then, pick up your right foot and rest it against your inner thigh.
3. Clasp your hands together and slowly raise them above your head, making sure that your pelvis is in a neutral position.

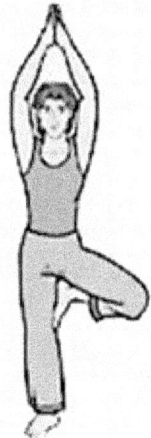

4. Hold this pose for as long as you can while taking deep, focused breaths (see Chapter 1 for additional breathing tips). It takes a while to get used to, but with continued practice you will be able to hold the pose for longer and longer.

The Warrior Pose

The warrior pose is a little simpler than the tree pose.

1. Spread your feet out so that they're about four feet apart.
2. Turn your head to the left, raising both of your arms outward so that they're parallel to the floor.
3. Shift your left foot ninety degrees to the left (it should be parallel to your line of sight) and slowly bend your knee forward. Hold this pose for as long as you can.

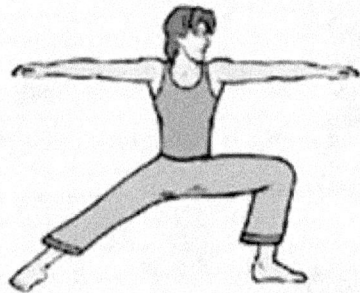

Cobra Pose

This exercise is designed to promote lower body flexibility. It is particularly beneficial to those with chronic lower back pain.

Unlike the other poses we've covered thus far, this one is done lying down.

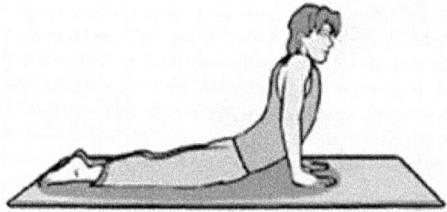

1. First, lie on your belly.
2. Raise your forehead and place your hands on either side of your chest, as if you were doing a push-up.
3. Straighten your arms until they stand perpendicular to the floor while moving your chest upward and outward. You should be feeling most of the strain in your lower back and abdomen.

Here are some wonderful exercises that combine posture, action and breath. They were developed by Dr. Stone, who continually refined his exercise programs for decades.

These exercises in particular show the importance of the fulcrum and leverage principle in Polarity Therapy. Note that "the feet are the basic fulcrum of the lowest level of precipitation, the emotionally chronic blocks in the water element of the body and also the earthly element of crystallization, inertia and solid waste blocks."

---

[1]Randolph Stone, Polarity Therapy Vol. I & Vol. II, CRCS PO Box 1460, Sebastopol, CA 95473

Health Posture with Up and Down Rocking Motion

This exercise is similar to a teeter totter and is helpful for relaxing muscles. It also has a stimulating effect through polarity function, from the negative to the positive side.

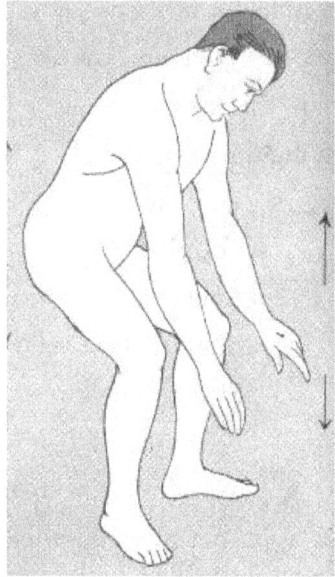

Figure 1

1. Assume a standing position pointing your toes outward so that your heels are about six inches apart while your toes are apart by about twice that.

2. Bend over slightly and bend your knees as in Figure 1.

3. Squat downward while making an up and down rocking motion as indicated by the arrows in Figure 1. Get down as far down as you can without straining or uncomfortably forcing your body (see Figure 2).

4. Hold the squat position with your armpits over your knees and your feet flat on the ground. Extend your arms outward for balance, but do not touch the floor.

5. Keeping your feet fully on the floor, rock forward and backward.

6. Change the rocking motion to a lateral one (from one side to the other).

7. Then, with a rocking motion similar to the lateral one above, twist your body so that you rotate around the center pivot of your spine.

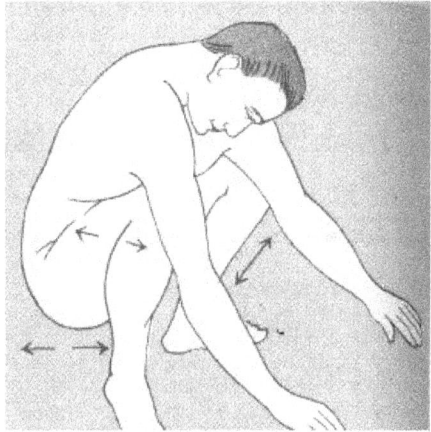

Figure 2

8. Remain in the squatting position and wrap your arms around your knees from the outside (see Figure 3). Make sure that you head is bent forward

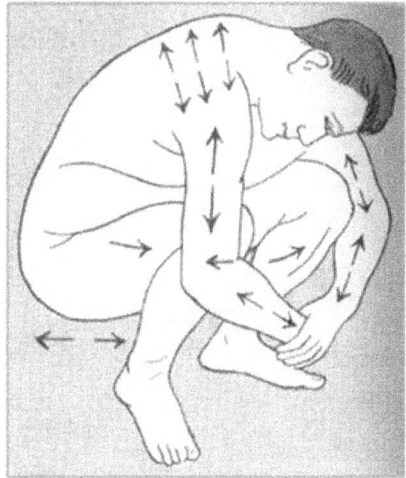

Figure 3

and your spine is extended. Your knees should be pushed together to stretch an entirely new set of muscles. Your hands should be in the locked position shown. The pull should be felt between your shoulders to be effective.

9. Rock back and forth, then from side to side. To finish, move the sacrum/pelvic area in a rocking motion lifting it slightly upwards, go back to the center and then lift it upwards on each side — as if you are on a swing. Remember this is a stretch and should feel playful rather than forced.

10. Then, with a rocking motion similar to the lateral one above, twist your body so that you rotate around the center pivot of your spine

11. When you stop rocking, take a deep breath and release it with a grunt. It is important that you end the exercise with the verbal sound.

The next set of exercises comes from Dr. Stone's *Health Building* book (sub title: The Conscious Art Of Living).

The Wood Chopper

This exercise also uses motion to integrate Life Energy with the action.

1. Stand with your feet relatively close together but not touching.

2.   Raise your arms over your head clasping your hands together and take a deep breath (see figure 4)

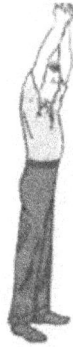

3.   Bend over until your clasped hands touch the inside of one leg just slightly above the ankle (figure 5). Put real effort behind the motion and, once your hands are on your leg, exhale and utter a "Ha" at the end of the exhalation (the sound should come automatically).

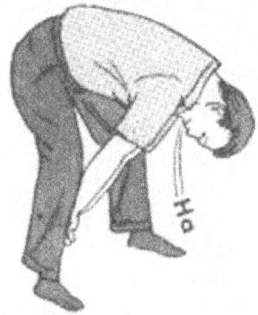

Figure 4 on the left, Figure 5 on the right

Vital Exercise with Natural Breath Expression

If you had trouble with the first exercise in this group, try this one instead. It doesn't require the rocking motions but still integrates Life Energy and works both your internal and external muscles. This exercise is often used for digestive disturbance and general sluggishness.

1.   Stand with your feet firmly on the floor. Let your head drop naturally.

2. Place your hands on bent knees and take a full deep breath through your nose.

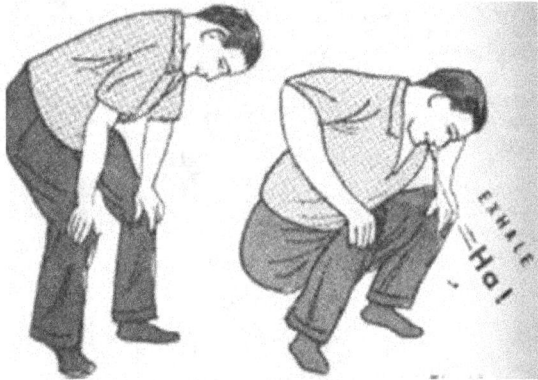

Figure 6 on the left, Figure 7 on the right

3. Bend over and drop down into a squatting position while exhaling forcefully and completely. As with the first exercise, you should naturally make a "Ha" sound.

Toning The Body

This exercise engages the Life Energy and most of the muscles in your body.

1. Stand with your legs wide apart and your hands on your knees (supporting the top of your body as if you are

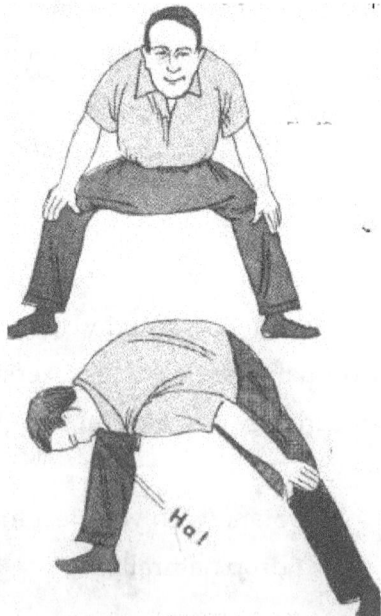

Figure 8 on top, Figure 9 below

66

ready to squat). As a reference point, it should feel as if there is an invisible chair behind you.

2. Balance yourself and take a deep breath through your nose, filling your diaphragm and belly with air, feeling the breath fill your body.

3. Hold to the count of five then exhale forcefully through your mouth, pulling in your belly as if to empty your belly from every bit of air.

4. Do this three to five times. As you do, your body will express a natural flow of energy which your muscles balance as a result.

5. Stay in this semi-squatting position; As you hold your 'stance' in this way (as in fig 8) breathing in deeply.

6. Holding the breath, move your body to the right and bend your upper body towards your right knee. As you lower the top half of your body it, release the breath with a loud HA!.

7. Go back to the semi squat position in Figure 8, breathe deeply and release the 'breath' with a loud HA!, this time leaning

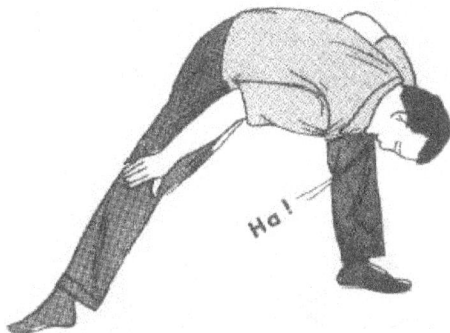

Figure 10

and releasing on the left (Figure 10).

8. Repeat these exercises five to six times each side with the <u>HA!</u> getting louder and more forceful each time. This will also release any anger or frustration you may be holding, thereby clearing the liver from any congested emotion.

Meditation

The term 'meditation' refers to a broad number of practices designed to clear the mind and promote relaxation. The texts of Buddhism, Sikhism, Christianity, Judaism, Wicca, Islam and Jainism all encourage meditation in some form. In the context of Hinduism (or, more specifically, yoga), meditation is used to unite yourself with the world around you, and to become one with nature. This is an important step towards achieving physical, mental and spiritual balance.

While you don't necessarily need to practice meditation in order to do yoga, it will help you get into the ideal state of mind. Yoga requires deep concentration and relaxation, and meditation helps you with both. If you can practice 'vision quest' exercises, meditation also helps you to reflect. Burning a perfumed stick or a fragrance oil of your chosen aroma is very helpful. Also, as you finish your meditation it can be beneficial to go into visualization mode. You can even use meditation to connect to the Law of Attraction.

wellbeing

balance

relaxation

concentration

strength

flexibility

meditation

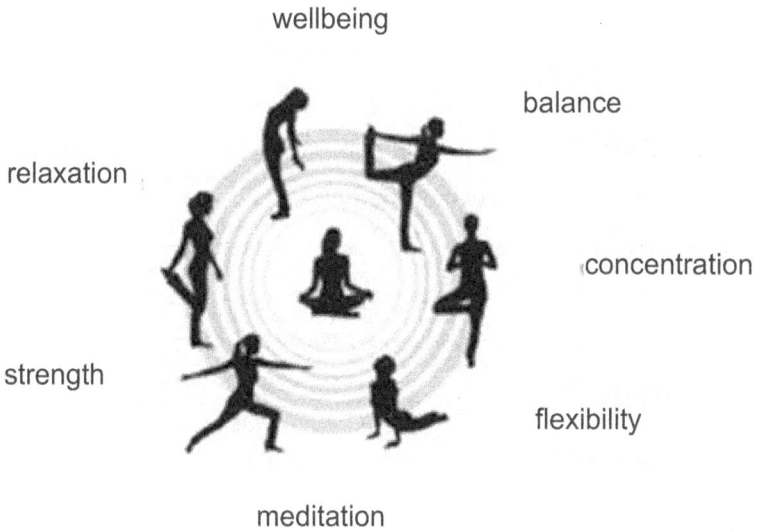

However, the act of clearing the mind is easier said than done, so here are some tips to help you get the most out of your time spent meditating.

Deepen Your Focus

One way to enter the optimal mindset for meditation is to focus your attention on one thing. This could mean repeating a mantra to yourself over and over again, visualizing a specific image in your head, or staring intently at an object in front of you (such as a lit candle). In any case, establish a point of focus and then concentrate all of your attention on that one point. The purpose of this exercise is to let this object consume you; become one with this object.

Sound

Chanting, either silently or out loud, is a powerful, effective way to enter a meditative state. Your mantra (the word or phrase that you chant) can be anything you want, but it should probably be something infused with personal meaning, like a prayer, an affirmation or a personal motto of yours. Remember, your aim is to focus your entire mind on this one phrase, so choose it accordingly.

Gazing

You can also choose to adopt a more visual-based method of focusing. To do this, keep your eyes open and concentrate your attention on a single object. Your point of focus can be absolutely anything. A lit candle is a popular point of focus for many yoga practitioners, but a statue, a painting, a flower or a mask would work just as well.

While concentration is important to this exercise, don't strain yourself. You should not be *leering* at the object; instead, opt for a soft, diffuse gaze. *Allow* your attention to hone in on the object, rather than forcing it. Imagine, if you will, that the object is a neighbor that you're welcoming into your mind. Let the object occupy your mind and consume your every thought until you and the object become one.

Note that these exercises are easier said than done, and they may not come naturally to you upon your first attempt. However, practice makes perfect, and in time the practice of meditation will be as natural to you as breathing.

Daily Schedule

Before each yoga exercise, you should take some time to meditate in order to enter the ideal mindset for practicing yoga. Do it for as long as it takes you to enter the meditative state. This may take a while at first, but it will take less and less time as you grow more experienced. Ideally, you should be practicing yoga for at least 30 minutes a day, not including the time you spend meditating beforehand. You should make sure that you're doing it in a distraction- free environment (for this reason, many people prefer to practice yoga in the evening, when they don't have other responsibilities to attend to).

At this point, you may feel overwhelmed. You may feel like the information provided to you thus far is too much to take in at once, and too much to keep track of on a daily basis. You may feel that the adoption of Dr. Stone's advice necessitates a radical lifestyle change; one that you're not willing to make.

However, there is no need to feel this way. The guidelines described in this book are meant to be adopted gradually, not immediately. You can begin by moderating your protein intake, and once you have the hang of that, you can start moderating your sodium intake, and then your carbohydrate intake, and so on and so forth.

If you don't feel comfortable doing yoga for 30 minutes a day, start out by doing it for, say, 10 minutes a day. The more you practice it, the more you'll enjoy it, and eventually you'll be willing to devote more and more of your schedule to it.

Also, not all of Dr. Stone's advice necessitates a major change in your life. According to him, there is one force that almost anyone can easily utilize to promote good health: the power of laughter.

The Laughter Cure

"Laughter is the language of the Gods and the tunes of Angels."
—Buddhist proverb

From time to time, you may hear someone claim that 'laughter is the best medicine.' You may be surprised to hear that this popular adage is not far from the truth. Hippocrates himself was a strong believer in the healing power of laughter, and like many of his other theories, his hypotheses regarding laughter were vindicated by the work of Dr. Stone and his colleagues.

Laughter helps trigger a number of different physical changes in the body. It can help alleviate stress, reduce tension, prevent heart disease, and even boost the effectiveness of your immune system. When you laugh or smile, your brain automatically thinks that you are happy and reacts accordingly.

In short, let your sense of humor shine. Allowing yourself to laugh (or even smile) more often will have a hugely beneficial effect on your physical, mental and spiritual health. Of all the advice you can take away from this book, this is arguably the most important. There's no treatment, natural or otherwise, that can substitute for a positive attitude and a smile in your heart. Check out a video on You Tube called "Contagious Subway Laughter" and start laughing more.

Chapter 7
WORKING WITH A POLARITY THERAPIST

Polarity Therapy is based on supporting the body's inherent self-healing intelligence and capabilities. It can take diverse forms, and is often very broad, making it a tool for health professionals in various therapeutic disciplines. It has strong connections to many other holistic health systems, both ancient and modern. Body energy fields are part of Ayurvedic tradition, and Polarity Therapy integrates the "Three Principles and Five Chakras."

Polarity practitioners use the natural phenomenon of repulsion/attraction (yin and yang) as a way of tracking energy flow and applying treatment to alleviate energy blockages or reverse energy direction.

What to Expect

In a typical session, your Polarity Therapist will gauge energetic attributes using observation, interview (in part to read the energy in your words and engage your emotions) and palpation methods. Energetic Touch will be a major treatment tool, with both soft and point-specific touch probably employed; associated contact will vary between light, medium and firm, but is almost always gentle. Rocking may be included.

Some of the techniques used are similar to those employed in reflexology, and some are derived from Osteopathy and Chiropractic (not surprising, given Dr. Stone's training). What makes the use of these techniques different in Polarity Therapy is that they are done with an energetic focus, rather than a manipulative one.

The therapist will also help you increase your self-awareness of subtle energetic sensations. These are often manifested as tingling, warmth or wavelike movement. You may exhibit emotional responses, like crying or laughing.

The results of Polarity Therapy sessions vary. You may experience profound relaxation or achieve an understanding of energetic patterns and their implications that will help empower you in terms of encouraging your body's ability to self-heal. It is not unusual to experience relief from anxiety attacks, breathing disorders and hypertension.

One of the most important things a Polarity Therapist will do is determine what the symptoms you may be experiencing indicate about your energy flow and recommend treatment and lifestyle changes to help alleviate the underlying problems. For example, headaches and migraines, as well as stomach cramps and other digestive disorders, can all be controlled or eliminated through Polarity Therapy. Likewise, back pain, general stress and other recurring conditions can be helped by this treatment modality.

A Polarity Therapist may also help you identify and treat 'energy cysts,' (stored emotions that are the result of a traumatic experience by placing your body in the same position it was at the time of your trauma.

Dietary advice will be given where necessary. This may include cleansing diets to rid the body of toxicity (procedures may also be applied). Additionally, a customized set of exercises may be recommended to support the bodywork that has been done during the session.

IN SUMMARY

The human body's extraordinary ability to heal itself remains largely untapped. People usually turn to traditional medicine like pills, surgery or other invasive procedures when they might easily be able to affect their own cure through proper eating, exercise, and meditation.

Eastern cultures have known since what seems like the beginning of time what Hippocrates, Dr. Stone and those practitioners of Polarity Therapy that followed Dr. Stone discovered —i.e., that proper use of elements from nature and body work like Polarity Therapy, Osteopathy, Chiropractics, Acupuncture and other alternative healing methods can be used to kick start the body's self-healing properties. Many of your daily aches and pains, digestive issues, feelings of lethargy and even emotional angst can be alleviated without the side effects and body trauma that can be associated with Western medicine. Polarity Therapy is based on the proven scientific discovery that the human body, like everything else on earth, is composed of energy and controlled by the positive and negative currents that flow throughout it. Physical and emotional issues occur when that polarity is disrupted and energy blockages are created. In addition to stretching and moving, Polarity Therapy, as practiced by a trained and experienced therapist, can release stuck patterns that block the energy flow. He or she can also recommend a healthy diet and exercises that will minimize problems or issues and stimulate your body's own healing properties.

It is essential that your Polarity Therapist be well versed in the teachings of Dr. Stone. Experience with other healing modalities is also a plus when choosing a therapist. If you would like to learn more about the benefits and processes of Polarity Therapy, or are looking for a therapist in the U.K., please feel free to email yotaloo@gmail.com or call Restore and Rejuvinate at ++44 1895 824 618.

GLOSSARY

ANS	Autonomic Nervous system
Ayurveda	Ancient Indian Medicine methods and modalities
CFS	Cerebral Spinal Fluid
Chiropractor	A trained health professional who uses a variety of non-surgical treatments, such as spinal manipulation and mobilization
Humors	A term used by Hippocrates to describe the elements: four in his time, five in Traditional Chinese Medicine (see below) and five in Polarity Therapy (see below)
Meditation	A practice of thinking or a state of consciousness
PNS	Parasympathetic nervous system
Polarity	The relationship between two opposite characteristics or tendencies. The polarity of the human body is based on the positive and negative currents of energy that flow throughout it.
Polarity Elements	Similar to Hippocrates humors, Fire, Air, Water, Earth and Ether

Neuroplasticity	The brain's ability to reorganize itself by forming new neural connections throughout life
Osteopath	A physician who bases diagnosis and treatment on the theory that the body's systems are interconnected. Osteopaths combine disease prevention and health maintenance with medicine, using a hands-on approach that may include massage or pressure points
SNS	Sympathetic nervous system
TCM	Traditional Chinese Medicine.
TCM Elements:	Fire: Small Intestine/Heart Earth: Stomach/Spleen, Metal: Large Intestine/Lungs, Water: Urinary Bladder/Kidney, Wood: Gall bladder/Liver:
Vegas nerve	Perhaps the longest nerve in the body, it connects the brain with most of your vital organs.
Yin	Female energy, night, dark, cold, weak etc.
Yang	Male energy, light, strong, hot, day etc.
Yoga	A Hindu spiritual and ascetic discipline, widely practiced for health and relaxation.

www.ingramcontent.com/pod-product-compliance
Lightning Source LLC
Chambersburg PA
CBHW070930270326
41927CB00011B/2803